WATER YOU WAITING FOR?

25 Ways Water Transforms Your Mind and Body

Asa Eccleston Kibilski

CONTENTS

H₂O: YOUR BODY'S BFF

Raise your glass (of water, that is!) to the most underrated superstar in the world of health and wellness: good old H_2O. Yes, we're talking about water, the liquid of life that you probably take for granted every single day. But what if I told you that this seemingly simple substance holds the power to transform your body, mind, and even your mood? Buckle up, because we're about to dive deep into the fascinating world of water and uncover why it's your body's absolute best friend.

Why Water Matters: More Than Just Quenching Your Thirst

Let's be real – water is more than just a way to avoid feeling parched on a hot day. It's the unsung hero behind countless bodily functions, working tirelessly behind the scenes to keep you feeling and looking your best. From your brain to your muscles, your skin to your gut, every single cell in your body relies on water to thrive. Think of it as the essential lubricant that keeps the gears of your life turning smoothly.

The Miracle Molecule: A Closer Look at H_2O

Water may be simple in its chemical composition – two hydrogen atoms bonded to one oxygen atom – but its impact on your body is anything but ordinary. This unassuming molecule plays a vital role in everything from temperature regulation to nutrient transport, waste removal to energy production. It's like the Swiss Army knife of your internal systems, ready to tackle any challenge that comes its way.

Water's Starring Roles: A Sneak Peek

In the following chapters, we'll delve deeper into the many ways water transforms your body and mind. Get ready to discover how water can:

- **Boost your brainpower:** Ever feel foggy or struggle to focus?

Water is your brain's best friend, helping it stay sharp and alert.

- **Amp up your mood:** Feeling blah? A few sips of water can lift your spirits and fight fatigue.
- **Give your skin a glow:** Forget expensive serums and creams – the secret to radiant skin might be as simple as drinking more water.
- **Detox your system:** Water helps flush out toxins, keeping your body running smoothly.
- **Support your weight loss goals:** By filling you up and suppressing your appetite, water can be a powerful tool in your weight loss arsenal.
- **Enhance your workouts:** Water helps your muscles perform at their best, whether you're a casual jogger or a seasoned athlete.

And that's just the tip of the iceberg! We'll also explore the surprising connection between water and your gut health, the importance of staying hydrated in hot weather, and even how water can save you money.

Ready to Dive In?

By now, you're probably realizing that water is much more than just a thirst quencher. It's the secret weapon you never knew you had, capable of transforming your health and well-being in countless ways. So, grab your favorite water bottle, fill it to the brim, and get ready to embark on a journey to discover the incredible power of H_2O. Your body will thank you!

THE SCIENCE OF HYDRATION – QUENCH YOUR THIRST, QUENCH YOUR CELLS

Alright, water enthusiasts, grab your favorite water bottle (and maybe a snack – this might get a little science-y) because we're about to dive headfirst into the fascinating world of hydration. Buckle up, because we're going to take a microscopic journey through your body to uncover the incredible ways water works its magic.

Hydration Highway: A Tour of Your Body's Waterways

Imagine your body as a bustling metropolis with a vast network of highways, roads, and alleyways. Water, in this analogy, is the lifeblood of this city, flowing through a complex system of pipes, tubes, and channels. These waterways, known as your circulatory and lymphatic systems, carry water to every nook and cranny of your body, ensuring that every cell receives the hydration it needs to thrive.

Water's Work Ethic: From Cells to Systems

Water isn't just a passive passenger on this journey – it's an active participant in countless bodily functions. Within your cells, water acts as a solvent, dissolving essential nutrients and transporting them to where they're needed most. It also helps regulate your body temperature, acting like a built-in air conditioner on hot days and a cozy blanket on cold ones. And let's not forget its role in waste removal – think of water as the sanitation crew that sweeps away cellular debris and keeps your system running smoothly.

The Osmosis Express: Water's Balancing Act

One of water's most impressive tricks is its ability to maintain balance within your body. Through a process called osmosis, water naturally flows from areas of low solute concentration (where there are fewer dissolved substances) to areas of high solute concentration. Think of it like a game of molecular tag – water molecules are constantly moving around, trying to even out the playing field. This balancing act is crucial for maintaining proper cell function and overall health.

Beyond the Basics: Water's Hidden Talents

But water's talents don't stop there. It also:

- **Lubricates your joints:** Water acts as a cushion and shock absorber, helping to prevent friction and wear and tear. So next time you're busting a move on the dance floor, thank water for keeping your joints happy.
- **Protects your organs and tissues:** Water forms a protective barrier around delicate structures like your brain and spinal cord, shielding them from injury.
- **Maintains blood volume:** Proper hydration is essential for maintaining a healthy blood volume, which in turn ensures efficient oxygen and nutrient delivery throughout your body.
- **Boosts energy production:** Water plays a crucial role in the production of ATP (adenosine triphosphate), the energy currency of your cells. So if you're feeling sluggish, grab a glass of water for a quick pick-me-up.

The Dehydration Downer: What Happens When You're Running on Empty

Now, let's flip the coin and see what happens when you don't drink enough water. Dehydration, the state of not having enough water in your body, can wreak havoc on your health and well-being. Symptoms can range from mild (dry mouth, thirst, fatigue) to severe (dizziness, confusion, heatstroke). Think of dehydration like a computer running low on battery power – everything starts to slow down, and eventually, the system crashes.

Stay Hydrated, Stay Happy

So, how can you ensure that your body's "waterworks" are functioning at their best? The answer is simple: drink plenty of water throughout the day. While there's no magic number, most adults should aim for at least eight 8-ounce glasses of water daily. But remember, your individual needs may vary depending on your activity level, climate, and overall health. Listen to your body's thirst cues and don't hesitate to reach for that water bottle whenever you need a refreshing refill.

The bottom line? Water is the unsung hero of your body's hydration story. By understanding the science behind how water works, you can empower yourself to make healthier choices and keep your body hydrated, happy, and thriving. So, raise a glass to the miracle molecule that keeps you going – your body will thank you for it!

WATER FUELS YOUR BRAIN – THINK SHARPER, FEEL STRONGER

Alright, fellow water warriors, get ready to embark on a mind-bending journey into the depths of your brain! We're about to uncover the fascinating relationship between water and cognitive function, and trust me, you'll never look at that glass of H_2O the same way again.

The Brain's Thirst for Knowledge (and Water)

Your brain, that three-pound marvel of neurons and synapses, is a thirsty beast. In fact, it's made up of about 75% water! Think of it as a high-performance machine that needs a constant supply of fuel to operate at its peak. Water, in this case, is the premium unleaded that keeps your mental engine humming along.

The Hydration-Cognition Connection: A Deeper Dive

So, how exactly does water impact your brainpower? The science is complex, but here's the gist:

1. **Electrical Conductivity:** Water is an excellent conductor of electricity, and your brain relies on electrical signals to transmit information. When you're properly hydrated, these signals zip along with lightning speed, allowing for quick thinking, sharp focus, and efficient problem-solving.

2. **Neurotransmitter Production:** Water is essential for the production of neurotransmitters, the chemical messengers that regulate your mood, emotions, and cognitive function. Without enough water, your brain's communication network can break down, leading to brain fog, irritability, and even depression.

3. **Blood Flow and Oxygen Delivery:** Water is a key component of blood, which carries oxygen and nutrients to your brain. When you're dehydrated, blood volume decreases, reducing the flow of oxygen to your brain cells. This can lead to fatigue, difficulty concentrating, and even headaches.
4. **Brain Volume:** Even mild dehydration can cause your brain to shrink temporarily! This might sound like something out of a sci-fi movie, but it's true. The good news is that rehydration quickly restores your brain to its normal size.

Dehydration: The Brain Drain

Think back to a time when you were really thirsty. Remember that feeling of fatigue, irritability, or difficulty focusing? That was your brain crying out for water! Even mild dehydration can negatively impact your cognitive function, including:

- **Decreased attention and focus:** Ever tried to read a page of text when you're parched? It's not easy, is it? Dehydration makes it harder to concentrate and pay attention to details.
- **Slower reaction times:** Need to make a quick decision? Dehydration can make your brain feel like it's stuck in molasses, slowing down your reaction time.
- **Impaired memory:** Trying to remember where you put your keys? If you're dehydrated, your brain might have a harder time retrieving memories.
- **Headaches and migraines:** For some people, dehydration can trigger headaches or migraines.

Hydrate for a Happy Head

The good news is that these effects are reversible! By simply drinking more water, you can replenish your brain's fuel supply and restore your cognitive function. Aim to drink water throughout the day, not just when you're thirsty. Keep a water bottle handy, set reminders on your phone, or even try infusing your water with fruits or herbs to make it more appealing.

Brain Food: Water and Beyond

While water is essential for optimal brain function, it's not the only factor to consider. A healthy diet, regular exercise, and sufficient sleep also play crucial roles in keeping your brain sharp. Think of water as the foundation upon which you build a healthy brain – it's the first step towards unlocking your full cognitive potential.

The Bottom Line

Your brain is a remarkable organ, capable of incredible feats of intelligence and creativity. But it needs your help to stay hydrated and perform at its best. So, next time you reach for a drink, make it water – your brain will thank you!

BOOST YOUR MOOD WITH H_2O - THE WATER-HAPPINESS CONNECTION

Ever notice how a glass of ice-cold water on a sweltering day can instantly lift your spirits? Or how a warm cup of herbal tea can soothe your soul on a gloomy afternoon? Well, it turns out there's more to this than just a refreshing sensation or a comforting ritual. Water, dear readers, has the power to influence your mood and emotional well-being in surprising ways. So, get ready to dive into the fascinating connection between hydration and happiness.

The Mood Molecule: Water's Role in Emotional Regulation

While it might sound a little woo-woo, water is essentially a mood molecule. It plays a crucial role in the production and balance of neurotransmitters, those chemical messengers that zip around your brain, regulating your emotions and mood. When you're properly hydrated, your brain is like a well-oiled machine, efficiently producing and utilizing neurotransmitters like serotonin (the "feel-good" chemical) and dopamine (the "reward" chemical).

But when you're dehydrated, even slightly, this delicate balance can be disrupted. Serotonin levels may dip, leaving you feeling down in the dumps, while dopamine production can stall, making it harder to experience pleasure and motivation. Think of it like a party in your brain where everyone's having a good time until the refreshments run out – things can get a little grumpy and chaotic.

Dehydration: The Mood Buster

So, what exactly does dehydration do to your mood? Here's a quick rundown of the not-so-fun effects:

- **Fatigue and irritability:** Ever snapped at your loved ones for no apparent reason? Dehydration can make you feel tired and irritable, even if you've gotten enough sleep.
- **Anxiety and depression:** Research suggests that even mild dehydration can worsen symptoms of anxiety and depression. So, if you're feeling blue, reaching for a glass of water might be a good first step.
- **Difficulty concentrating and remembering:** Remember that brain fog we talked about earlier? Dehydration can make it even harder to focus and recall information.
- **Low mood and negative emotions:** When you're dehydrated, your brain is more likely to perceive situations as stressful or threatening, leading to feelings of negativity and pessimism.

Hydrate for Happiness: Water's Mood-Boosting Benefits

The good news is that these negative effects are reversible! By simply increasing your water intake, you can replenish your brain's supply of mood-boosting neurotransmitters and experience a noticeable shift in your emotional well-being. Here's how water can lift your spirits:

- **Increased energy and alertness:** Water helps your body produce ATP, the energy currency of your cells. More energy equals more vitality and a brighter outlook on life.
- **Reduced stress and anxiety:** Studies have shown that staying hydrated can lower cortisol levels, the stress hormone that can wreak havoc on your mood.
- **Improved mood and positive emotions:** When you're well-hydrated, your brain is better equipped to handle challenges and cope with stress, leading to a more positive outlook.
- **Enhanced cognitive function:** Remember, water fuels your brain! When your brain is hydrated, it's easier to focus, think clearly, and make decisions.

Hydration Habits for a Happier You

So, how can you make hydration a regular part of your mood-boosting routine? Here are a few tips:

- **Keep water within reach:** Carry a reusable water bottle with you and refill it throughout the day.
- **Make it tasty:** If plain water isn't your thing, try infusing it with fruits, herbs, or cucumbers for a refreshing twist.
- **Set reminders:** Use an app or set alarms on your phone to remind you to drink water regularly.
- **Listen to your body:** Pay attention to your thirst cues – they're your body's way of telling you it needs a hydration boost.

Remember, water isn't just a thirst quencher – it's a mood enhancer, a stress reducer, and a cognitive booster. So, drink up and let the happiness flow!

CLEAR SKIN, CLEAR MIND: WATER'S BEAUTY BENEFITS

Ladies and gentlemen, it's time for a glow-up! But before you reach for that expensive serum or face mask, let's talk about the simplest, most affordable beauty elixir out there: water. Yes, that's right – good old H_2O is not just essential for your overall health, but it also plays a starring role in giving you that coveted radiant complexion. So, grab your water bottle (and maybe a mirror) as we delve into the fascinating connection between hydration and your skin's natural beauty.

The Skin You're In: Your Body's Largest Organ

Let's start with a quick biology lesson: your skin is your body's largest organ, acting as a protective barrier against the elements while also playing a crucial role in temperature regulation, sensation, and immune function. But it's not just a shield – your skin is a reflection of your inner health. And when it comes to keeping your skin healthy and glowing, hydration is key.

Water Works: Hydration's Role in Skin Health

Think of your skin cells like tiny grapes. When they're plump and hydrated, they look firm, smooth, and radiant. But when they're dehydrated, they shrivel up like raisins, leading to a dull, lackluster complexion. Water helps maintain your skin's elasticity and plumpness by providing essential moisture to the cells. It also helps flush out toxins and impurities that can clog pores and contribute to breakouts.

Beyond Beauty: Water's Other Skin Benefits

But water's benefits for your skin go beyond mere aesthetics. Here are a few more ways hydration can improve your skin health:

- **Reduced wrinkles and fine lines:** Proper hydration can help plump up the skin, minimizing the appearance of fine lines and wrinkles.

- **Improved elasticity:** Hydrated skin is more resilient and less prone to sagging or stretching.
- **Faster wound healing:** Water is essential for cell regeneration, which is crucial for healing cuts, scrapes, and other skin injuries.
- **Reduced inflammation:** Dehydration can trigger inflammation, which can contribute to skin conditions like eczema and psoriasis.
- **Protection from environmental damage:** Well-hydrated skin is better equipped to protect itself from environmental stressors like pollution and UV radiation.

Dehydrated Skin: A Recipe for Disaster

On the flip side, dehydration can wreak havoc on your skin. When you're not drinking enough water, your skin cells become depleted, leading to a host of undesirable side effects:

- **Dryness and flakiness:** Dehydrated skin can feel rough, tight, and itchy.
- **Dullness and uneven tone:** Lack of moisture can make your skin look dull and lifeless.
- **Increased oil production:** Ironically, dehydrated skin can actually produce more oil, leading to clogged pores and breakouts.
- **Accelerated aging:** Dehydration can contribute to premature wrinkles and fine lines.
- **Increased sensitivity:** Dehydrated skin is more prone to irritation and allergic reactions.

Hydrate for a Healthy Glow: Tips for Radiant Skin

Ready to unleash your skin's natural glow? Here are a few hydration tips to keep your complexion looking its best:

- **Drink up:** Aim for at least eight 8-ounce glasses of water per day. You can also get hydration from water-rich fruits and vegetables like watermelon, cucumbers, and berries.

- **Moisturize:** Apply a good moisturizer after cleansing to lock in hydration.
- **Humidify:** Use a humidifier in dry environments to add moisture to the air and prevent your skin from drying out.
- **Protect your skin:** Wear sunscreen daily to protect your skin from harmful UV rays, which can accelerate aging and damage your skin.
- **Get enough sleep:** Sleep is essential for skin repair and regeneration. Aim for 7-8 hours of quality sleep each night.

Remember, healthy skin starts from the inside out. By prioritizing hydration, you can nourish your skin cells, promote a radiant complexion, and even slow down the aging process. So, raise a glass of water to your skin's health – it's the most natural (and affordable!) beauty treatment you can give yourself.

THE NATURAL DETOX: WATER'S ROLE IN FLUSHING OUT TOXINS

Welcome to the detoxification station, folks! No, we're not talking about those trendy juice cleanses or questionable herbal supplements. We're diving into the world of your body's most natural and effective detoxifier: water. That's right, the humble H_2O is more than just a thirst quencher – it's your body's built-in sanitation crew, working tirelessly to remove waste and keep your system running smoothly.

Your Body's Waste Management System: A Symphony of Organs

Before we get into water's starring role in this detoxification drama, let's take a quick tour of your body's waste management system. It's a complex symphony of organs, each with its unique role to play:

- **Liver:** Your liver is like the diligent factory worker, filtering your blood, breaking down toxins, and transforming them into less harmful substances.
- **Kidneys:** These bean-shaped powerhouses are the filtration experts, removing waste products from your blood and producing urine.
- **Lungs:** While primarily responsible for respiration, your lungs also help expel certain waste products, like carbon dioxide, through your breath.
- **Skin:** Your skin, the body's largest organ, plays a role in detoxification through sweat. It's like a mini sauna, releasing toxins along with excess water and salts.

Water's Role: The Ultimate Flush

Now, where does water fit into this intricate system? Think of water as the delivery truck that picks up waste from your cells and transports it to the organs responsible for disposal. Without enough water, this system can slow down or even break down, leading to a buildup of toxins in your body.

Water's detoxifying powers come into play in several ways:

1. **Kidney Function:** Water is essential for kidney function, helping them filter waste products from your blood and produce urine. When you're dehydrated, your kidneys have to work harder to do their job, which can put a strain on your system.
2. **Liver Function:** Water helps your liver metabolize and eliminate toxins more efficiently. It also aids in the production of bile, a substance that helps break down fats and remove waste products from your digestive system.
3. **Bowel Movements:** Water helps keep your stool soft and easy to pass, preventing constipation and promoting regular bowel movements. This is crucial for eliminating waste products from your body.
4. **Sweat Production:** Water is a key component of sweat, which helps your body release toxins through your skin. So, next time you're breaking a sweat at the gym, remember that you're also giving your body a natural detox.

The Dehydration Dilemma: A Toxic Buildup

When you're not drinking enough water, your body's detoxification system can't function optimally. Waste products can build up in your system, leading to a variety of unpleasant symptoms:

- **Fatigue:** Your body has to work harder to eliminate toxins when you're dehydrated, which can leave you feeling tired and sluggish.
- **Headaches:** Toxins can irritate your brain and trigger headaches.
- **Skin problems:** Dehydration can lead to dry, dull skin, and

even acne breakouts.

- **Constipation:** Lack of water can make it difficult to have regular bowel movements, leading to a buildup of waste products in your colon.

Hydrate for Detoxification: The Natural Solution

The good news is that you can easily support your body's natural detoxification process by simply drinking more water. Aim for at least eight 8-ounce glasses of water per day, and more if you're active or live in a hot climate. You can also boost your water intake by eating hydrating fruits and vegetables like watermelon, cucumbers, and spinach.

Remember, water is your body's best friend when it comes to detoxification. It's a natural, affordable, and effective way to flush out toxins and keep your system running smoothly. So, raise a glass to your health – and to your body's incredible ability to cleanse itself!

WATER FOR WEIGHT LOSS – THE WEIGHT-LOSS WONDER

Alright, water warriors, it's time to tackle a topic that's probably on a lot of our minds: weight loss. Now, before you roll your eyes and think, "Oh great, another water cure-all," let me assure you that this isn't some fad diet or quick fix. Instead, we're going to delve into the fascinating and scientifically-backed ways that water can genuinely support your weight loss goals. Get ready to discover how this humble liquid can become your secret weapon in the battle of the bulge.

The H_2O-Weight Loss Connection: Not Magic, Just Science

Let's be clear: water alone isn't going to magically melt away pounds. But it can play a significant role in your weight loss journey, and the science behind it is pretty fascinating. Here's how water can give your weight loss efforts a boost:

1. Calorie-Free Cravings Crusher: Let's face it, we often mistake thirst for hunger. That rumbling tummy might be your body asking for water, not a snack. By reaching for a glass of water first, you can avoid unnecessary calories and help control your appetite.

2. The Natural Appetite Suppressant: Ever notice how a big glass of water before a meal can make you feel fuller faster? Water takes up space in your stomach, sending signals to your brain that you're satisfied. This can help you eat less and ultimately consume fewer calories.

3. Metabolism Booster: Studies have shown that drinking water can temporarily increase your metabolism, the rate at which your body burns calories. This effect is more pronounced with cold water, as your body has to work harder to warm it up to body temperature. While it's not a massive calorie burn, every little bit helps,

right?

4. The Workout Wingman: Proper hydration is essential for optimal exercise performance. When you're well-hydrated, you'll have more energy, endurance, and stamina, allowing you to work out harder and longer, ultimately burning more calories.

Water's Weight-Loss Wonders: Real-World Results

Don't just take my word for it – research has shown that increasing water intake can lead to significant weight loss results. A study published in the journal Obesity found that overweight and obese adults who increased their water intake by 1 liter per day lost an average of 4.4 pounds over 12 weeks – without making any other changes to their diet or exercise routine!

Another study found that drinking water before meals can help reduce calorie intake and promote weight loss. Participants who drank 500ml of water 30 minutes before each meal lost 44% more weight over 12 weeks compared to those who didn't.

Tips for Hydrating Your Way to Weight Loss

Ready to make water your weight loss BFF? Here are a few tips to get you started:

- Drink a glass of water before each meal: This will help you feel fuller and eat less.
- Carry a water bottle with you: Make it a habit to sip on water throughout the day.
- Set reminders: Use an app or set alarms to remind you to drink water regularly.
- Flavor your water: If plain water is boring, try infusing it with fruits, herbs, or cucumbers.
- Track your water intake: There are many apps available to help you monitor your daily water consumption.

A Word of Caution: Water is Not a Miracle Cure

While water can be a powerful tool for weight loss, it's important to remember that it's not a magic bullet. Sustainable weight loss requires a combination of healthy eating habits, regular exercise, and lifestyle changes. But by incorporating water into your daily routine, you can give your weight loss efforts a significant boost and enjoy the numerous other benefits this amazing liquid has to offer.

So, drink up, water warriors! Your body (and your waistline) will thank you for it.

BEAT THE HEAT WITH HYDRATION - WATER'S COOLING SUPERPOWERS

Welcome to the splash zone, water warriors! It's time to crank up the heat (literally) and explore the incredible ways water helps you chill out when the temperature rises. Whether you're a sun-worshipper, an outdoor enthusiast, or someone who simply melts in the summer heat, this chapter is your ultimate guide to staying cool, calm, and hydrated under the scorching sun.

The Human Radiator: How Your Body Beats the Heat

Before we dive into water's role in this process, let's take a quick look at how your body naturally regulates its temperature. Think of yourself as a finely tuned radiator, constantly adjusting to maintain a comfortable internal temperature of around 98.6°F (37°C). When you get too hot, your body has a few tricks up its sleeve to cool down:

1. Sweat It Out: Your sweat glands kick into high gear, releasing sweat onto your skin. As the sweat evaporates, it takes heat with it, cooling you down like a natural air conditioner. Pretty clever, huh?
2. Blood Vessel Expansion: Your blood vessels near the skin's surface dilate (widen), allowing more blood to flow close to the skin and release heat into the environment. It's like opening the windows to let a cool breeze in.
3. Increased Respiration: You might notice yourself breathing faster when you're hot. This is your body's way of expelling excess heat through your breath.

Water's Role: The Coolant of Life

Now, where does water come into play? Think of water as the coolant that keeps your body's radiator running smoothly. It's essential for all three of the cooling mechanisms we just discussed:

- Sweat Production: Without enough water, your body can't produce enough sweat to effectively cool you down. Imagine trying to run your air conditioner without any refrigerant – it's just not going to work.
- Blood Volume: Water is a major component of blood, and maintaining adequate blood volume is crucial for transporting heat away from your core to your skin's surface.
- Hydration and Breathing: Staying hydrated helps keep your respiratory system moist, allowing you to breathe easily and expel excess heat through your breath.

Dehydration Dangers: When Your Body Overheats

When you don't drink enough water, your body's ability to regulate temperature is compromised. This can lead to dehydration, which can quickly escalate from mild discomfort to a dangerous condition. Here are some signs of dehydration to watch out for:

- Thirst (duh!): This is your body's most obvious signal that it needs more fluids.
- Dry mouth and throat: When you're dehydrated, your saliva production decreases, leading to a dry, sticky feeling in your mouth.
- Dark urine: If your pee is a deep yellow or amber color, it's a sign that you need to drink more water.
- Fatigue and dizziness: Dehydration can make you feel tired, weak, and lightheaded.
- Muscle cramps: Lack of water can cause your muscles to cramp up, especially during exercise.

In severe cases, dehydration can lead to heat exhaustion or heatstroke, which are medical emergencies and require immediate attention.

Hydration Heroes: Tips for Staying Cool and Hydrated

Ready to beat the heat and keep your cool? Here are some hydration tips for hot weather:

- Drink water regularly: Don't wait until you're thirsty to drink. Aim to sip on water throughout the day, especially if you're active or spending time outdoors.
- Electrolyte boost: If you're sweating a lot, consider adding electrolytes to your water to replenish lost minerals like sodium and potassium.
- Eat your water: Water-rich fruits and vegetables like watermelon, cucumbers, and berries can help you stay hydrated while providing essential nutrients.
- Cool down from the inside out: Enjoy chilled beverages like iced tea, infused water, or even a popsicle to help lower your body temperature.
- Limit alcohol and caffeine: These beverages can actually dehydrate you, so enjoy them in moderation, especially in hot weather.

Remember, water is your body's best friend when it comes to beating the heat. So, drink up, stay hydrated, and enjoy those sunny days without feeling like a melted popsicle.

JOINT JUICE - HOW WATER LUBRICATES AND PROTECTS YOUR JOINTS

Alright, water warriors, it's time to get moving! We're about to delve into the fascinating world of joints, those remarkable hinges that allow us to bend, twist, and groove our way through life. But before you break out your best dance moves, let's talk about the unsung hero that keeps your joints healthy and happy: water. Yes, that's right – good old H_2O is not just for quenching your thirst, it's also essential for keeping your joints lubricated and pain-free.

Joint Anatomy 101: A Quick Refresher

Before we dive into the nitty-gritty of how water works its magic on your joints, let's do a quick anatomy refresher. Your joints are where two or more bones meet, and they come in various shapes and sizes, from the hinge joint in your elbow to the ball-and-socket joint in your shoulder. Each joint is surrounded by a capsule filled with synovial fluid, a thick, slippery liquid that acts as a lubricant and shock absorber. Think of it like the WD-40 of your body, keeping your joints moving smoothly and preventing painful friction.

Water's Role: The Joint Juice

Now, where does water come into play? Well, synovial fluid is primarily made up of water! It's like a water balloon for your joints, providing the cushioning and lubrication they need to glide effortlessly through their range of motion. Without enough water, synovial fluid can become thick and sticky, leading to stiffness, pain, and even joint damage.

Think of your joints like a well-oiled machine – if you don't keep it lubricated, the parts will start to grind together, causing friction and wear and tear. The same goes for your joints – without adequate water, they can become dry, creaky, and prone to injury.

The Dehydration Dilemma: Dry Joints, Achy Days

When you're dehydrated, your body starts to prioritize its water resources, and your joints are often the first to suffer. The synovial fluid becomes less viscous and less effective at lubricating the joint, leading to increased friction and inflammation. This can manifest as stiffness, pain, and a limited range of motion.

Imagine trying to ride a bike with rusty, squeaky gears – it's not a pleasant experience, is it? The same goes for your joints – when they're not properly lubricated, movement becomes difficult and painful.

Hydration for Happy Joints: Drink Up for Smooth Moves

The good news is that you can easily protect your joints and keep them moving freely by simply staying hydrated. Here's how water benefits your joints:

- **Lubrication:** Water is the main component of synovial fluid, which acts as a lubricant for your joints.
- **Shock Absorption:** Water helps cushion your joints, protecting them from impact and wear and tear.
- **Nutrient Delivery:** Water helps transport essential nutrients to your cartilage, the smooth tissue that covers the ends of your bones and allows them to glide smoothly against each other.
- **Waste Removal:** Water helps flush out waste products that can build up in your joints and contribute to inflammation.

Hydration Tips for Healthy Joints:

Ready to give your joints the TLC they deserve? Here are a few tips to keep them hydrated and happy:

- **Drink up:** Aim for at least eight 8-ounce glasses of water per day. You can also get hydration from water-rich fruits and vegetables like watermelon, cucumbers, and berries.

- **Move your body:** Regular exercise helps to pump synovial fluid into your joints, keeping them lubricated and healthy.
- **Warm up before exercise:** Start your workouts with gentle movements to get your joints moving and increase blood flow.
- **Listen to your body:** If you experience joint pain, stop and rest. Don't push through the pain, as this can worsen the problem.

Remember, your joints are designed to move, and water is the key to keeping them moving smoothly and pain-free. So, raise a glass to your joints – and to the miracle molecule that keeps them lubricated and happy!

PEAK PERFORMANCE WITH H$_2$O - THE WORKOUT WINGMAN

Water warriors, it's time to lace up your sneakers, grab your water bottle, and hit the gym (or the park, or the trail, or wherever your workout takes you). We're about to uncover the fascinating relationship between hydration and exercise performance, and trust me, you won't want to leave home without your trusty H$_2$O sidekick ever again.

The Exercise-Hydration Equation: Fueling Your Fitness

Whether you're a casual jogger, a weekend warrior, or a hardcore athlete, your body relies on water to perform at its best during exercise. Think of water as the high-octane fuel that powers your muscles, regulates your temperature, and keeps your mind sharp when the going gets tough. Without enough water, your workouts can suffer, and you might not be able to reach your full potential.

How Dehydration Hinders Your Workouts

Dehydration is like a wrench in the gears of your exercise machine. It can lead to a host of performance-sapping effects, including:

- **Decreased Endurance:** When you're dehydrated, your blood volume drops, making it harder for your heart to pump blood and oxygen to your working muscles. This can lead to fatigue, weakness, and a shortened workout.
- **Muscle Cramps:** Dehydration can also trigger muscle cramps, those painful involuntary contractions that can sideline you in the middle of a workout.
- **Elevated Heart Rate:** Your heart has to work harder to circulate less blood volume when you're dehydrated, leading to a higher heart rate and potentially putting extra strain on your cardiovascular system.

- **Reduced Cognitive Function:** Dehydration can impair your brain's ability to focus, make decisions, and react quickly, which can be dangerous during certain activities.
- **Increased Perceived Exertion:** When you're dehydrated, even moderate exercise can feel more challenging, making it harder to push yourself and reach your goals.

Hydration Hacks for Peak Performance

Ready to take your workouts to the next level? Here are a few hydration tips to optimize your exercise performance:

1. Pre-Workout Hydration: Start hydrating well before your workout. Aim to drink 16-20 ounces of water in the two hours leading up to your exercise session.
2. Sip and Sweat: During your workout, sip on water regularly to replenish fluids lost through sweat. A good rule of thumb is to drink 7-10 ounces every 10-20 minutes of exercise.
3. Post-Workout Rehydration: After your workout, continue to drink water to rehydrate and replenish electrolytes lost through sweat. You can also opt for a sports drink containing electrolytes like sodium and potassium.

Customizing Your Hydration Strategy:

Your individual hydration needs will vary depending on a few factors:

- **Intensity and Duration of Exercise:** The harder and longer you exercise, the more water you'll need.
- **Climate and Environment:** Hot and humid weather can increase your sweat rate, requiring you to drink more fluids.
- **Individual Factors:** Your body size, sweat rate, and overall health can also influence your hydration needs.

Listen to Your Body: Thirst is Your Guide

While these guidelines are a good starting point, it's important to listen to your body's thirst cues. Thirst is your body's way of telling you it needs more fluids. Don't ignore it! If you're feeling thirsty, drink up.

Water: The MVP of Your Workout

Whether you're a seasoned athlete or a casual exerciser, water is the MVP of your workout routine. It's the natural, affordable, and effective way to fuel your performance, prevent dehydration, and help you reach your fitness goals. So, raise a glass (or bottle) to your health – and to the incredible power of H_2O!

WATER WORKS: THE GUT-BRAIN CONNECTION AND DIGESTIVE HEALTH

Alright, water warriors, prepare to embark on a journey to the center of your gut! No, we're not talking about a thrill ride at the amusement park – we're diving into the fascinating connection between water and your digestive system. Get ready to discover how this humble liquid plays a starring role in keeping your gut happy, healthy, and humming along smoothly.

The Gut: Your Second Brain

Before we get into the nitty-gritty of how water affects your gut, let's take a moment to appreciate this incredible organ. Your gut, also known as your gastrointestinal tract, is responsible for more than just digesting your food. It's home to trillions of bacteria, collectively known as your gut microbiome, which play a crucial role in your overall health and well-being.

In fact, scientists have dubbed the gut your "second brain" because it has its own nervous system, produces neurotransmitters (those chemical messengers that regulate your mood and emotions), and even communicates with your "first" brain through a complex network of nerves. It's like a bustling metropolis, with trillions of tiny residents working together to keep you healthy and happy.

Water's Role in Gut Health: The Digestive Dynamo

So, where does water fit into this gutsy ecosystem? Well, it turns out that water is essential for every step of the digestive process, from the moment you take your first bite to the, well, let's just say the final result.

1. Saliva Power: The digestive process begins in your mouth, where saliva (which is mostly water) helps break

down food and prepare it for its journey down your esophagus.

2. Esophageal Ease: Water helps lubricate your esophagus, making it easier for food to slide down smoothly. Without enough water, you might experience that dreaded feeling of food getting stuck.

3. Stomach Churn: Water helps create the stomach acid necessary for breaking down food and killing harmful bacteria. It also helps churn and mix the food with digestive enzymes, creating a soupy mixture called chyme.

4. Intestinal Flow: Water is essential for maintaining proper bowel function. It helps keep your stool soft and easy to pass, preventing constipation and promoting regular bowel movements. Think of it as the WD-40 of your digestive system, keeping things moving along smoothly.

5. Gut Microbiome Balance: Water helps create the ideal environment for your gut bacteria to thrive. A healthy gut microbiome is crucial for digestion, immune function, and even mental health.

Dehydration: A Gut-Wrenching Experience

When you're not drinking enough water, your digestive system can throw a tantrum. Dehydration can lead to a host of uncomfortable and even painful digestive issues, including:

- Constipation: This is one of the most common side effects of dehydration. When you're not drinking enough water, your stool can become hard and difficult to pass.

- Indigestion and Heartburn: Dehydration can decrease the production of stomach acid, making it harder to digest food and leading to indigestion and heartburn.

- Bloating and Gas: Dehydration can disrupt the balance of bacteria in your gut, leading to an overgrowth of gas-producing bacteria and causing bloating and discomfort.

- Stomach Pains and Cramps: Dehydration can trigger spasms in your intestines, leading to painful cramps.

Hydrate for a Happy Gut: The Digestive Elixir

The good news is that you can easily soothe your gut and keep it happy by simply drinking more water. Aim for at least eight 8-ounce glasses of water per day, and more if you're active or eating a high-fiber diet. You can also get hydration from water-rich fruits and vegetables like watermelon, cucumbers, and celery.

Remember, your gut is like a second brain, and it needs water to function properly. So, drink up and let your gut do its happy dance!

BEYOND THIRST: HIDDEN SIGNS OF DEHYDRATION YOU MIGHT BE MISSING

Alright, water warriors, it's time for a dehydration detective mission! While thirst is the most obvious sign your body needs more H_2O, it's not always the first clue. In fact, there are several sneaky signs of dehydration lurking beneath the surface, disguised as everyday annoyances or minor health complaints. So, grab your magnifying glass (and your water bottle) as we uncover these hidden signs and learn how to outsmart dehydration before it derails your day.

The Dehydration Disguise: More Than Just a Dry Mouth

Think of dehydration as a master of disguise, cleverly concealing its true identity behind a variety of seemingly unrelated symptoms. It's like a chameleon, blending into its surroundings and making it difficult to spot until it's too late. But fear not, water warriors, we're about to expose this sly culprit's tricks.

1. The Foggy Brain: Can't remember where you put your keys? Struggling to focus on a task? It might not just be a case of "mommy brain" or a Monday morning slump. Dehydration can impair cognitive function, leading to brain fog, forgetfulness, and difficulty concentrating. So, before you blame your memory lapse on aging, try chugging a glass of water and see if that clears the fog.

2. The Crankypants: Feeling irritable, moody, or just plain grumpy? Don't be so quick to blame your hormones or your boss. Dehydration can mess with your mood, making you more prone to irritability, anxiety, and even anger. Next time you're feeling like a bear with a sore

head, try reaching for a water bottle instead of a stress ball.

3. The Achy Breaky Body: Muscle cramps, headaches, and joint pain? Before you pop a painkiller, consider whether dehydration might be the culprit. Lack of water can lead to muscle cramps, trigger headaches, and even worsen joint pain due to decreased lubrication. So, before you reach for the medicine cabinet, try hydrating first.

4. The Hunger Games: Feeling hungry even though you just ate? Your stomach might be growling for water, not food. Dehydration can mimic hunger signals, leading to unnecessary snacking and potential weight gain. Next time your tummy rumbles, try drinking a glass of water and see if that satisfies your cravings.

5. The Bathroom Blues: Constipation, anyone? Dehydration is a common cause of constipation, as it can make your stool hard and difficult to pass. If you're struggling with irregularity, increasing your water intake can help get things moving again.

6. The Skin Snitch: Your skin is a telltale sign of your hydration status. Dry, flaky, or itchy skin? Dehydration could be the culprit. When your body lacks water, your skin loses its natural moisture and elasticity, leading to a dull, lifeless complexion.

7. The Dark Side: Is your pee looking a little too yellow? That's a surefire sign of dehydration. When you're well-hydrated, your urine should be pale yellow or almost clear. Darker urine indicates that your kidneys are working overtime to conserve water, which is not a good thing.

Decoding Dehydration: Your Body's Secret Language

By paying attention to these subtle signs of dehydration, you can take action before it becomes a bigger problem. Remember, your body is constantly communicating with you. All you have to do is listen and respond with a refreshing glass of H_2O.

HOW MUCH WATER DO YOU REALLY NEED? – THE HYDRATION CALCULATOR

Alright, water warriors, it's time to crunch some numbers! We've talked about the countless ways water benefits your body and mind, but the burning question remains: how much water do you *really* need to drink each day? Is it the classic "8 glasses a day" rule, or is there more to it? Grab your calculators (or just your water bottle – we'll do the math for you) as we dive into the fascinating world of hydration calculations and personalized water needs.

The 8x8 Rule: Myth or Magic?

Let's start by addressing the elephant in the room: the "8x8 rule," which recommends drinking eight 8-ounce glasses of water per day. While it's a catchy phrase and a good starting point for many people, it's not a one-size-fits-all solution. Your individual water needs can vary depending on several factors, including your:

- **Body size and composition:** Larger individuals generally need more water than smaller individuals. Muscle tissue also holds more water than fat tissue, so athletes and those with higher muscle mass may need to increase their intake.
- **Activity level:** If you're sweating buckets at the gym or simply moving around a lot, you'll need to replenish those lost fluids.
- **Climate and environment:** Hot and humid weather can increase your sweat rate, requiring you to drink more water to stay hydrated.
- **Overall health:** Certain medical conditions, medications, and dietary factors can affect your fluid needs.

The Personalized Hydration Equation: Factors to Consider

So, how can you determine your personal water needs? Here are a few factors to consider:

1. Thirst: Your body's thirst mechanism is a pretty reliable indicator of when you need to drink. Pay attention to those thirst cues and don't hesitate to reach for your water bottle when you feel parched.

2. Urine Color: Another way to gauge your hydration status is by looking at your pee. Ideally, your urine should be pale yellow or almost clear. If it's dark yellow or amber, it's a sign you need to drink more water.

3. Activity Level: If you're physically active, you'll need to drink more water to replace fluids lost through sweat. A good rule of thumb is to drink an additional 1.5-2.5 cups of water for every hour of exercise.

4. Climate: Hot and humid weather can increase your sweat rate, so be sure to drink more water when the temperature rises. If you're traveling to a different climate, adjust your water intake accordingly.

5. Individual Needs: Certain medical conditions, medications, and dietary factors can affect your fluid needs. If you have any concerns, talk to your doctor or a registered dietitian to determine your individual hydration requirements.

The Hydration Calculator: Doing the Math

Now, let's get down to the nitty-gritty of calculating your personalized water intake. Here's a simple formula you can use:

- Take your body weight in pounds and divide it by two. This number is the minimum amount of water you should drink in ounces per day.

- Add 12 ounces of water for every 30 minutes of exercise.

For example, if you weigh 150 pounds and exercise for 60 minutes a day, you should aim to drink at least 105 ounces of water daily.

Remember, this is just a starting point. You might need to adjust your intake based on your individual needs and the factors mentioned earlier. And if you're ever unsure, don't hesitate to consult with a healthcare professional for personalized guidance.

Hydration: A Balancing Act

Just like Goldilocks, you want to find the "just right" amount of water for your body. Too little can lead to dehydration, while too much can dilute your electrolytes and potentially cause hyponatremia, a rare but serious condition. The key is to listen to your body, pay attention to your urine color, and adjust your water intake as needed.

Hydration is a journey, not a destination. It's about finding what works best for you and making water a consistent part of your daily routine. So, raise a glass to your health – and to the personalized hydration plan that keeps you feeling your best!

HYDRATION MYTHS BUSTED – SEPARATING FACT FROM FICTION

Alright, water warriors, it's time to put on our detective hats and bust some hydration myths! Like any popular topic, the world of water and hydration is awash with misinformation, half-truths, and downright wacky claims. So, grab your water bottle (filled with actual water, not unicorn tears) as we separate fact from fiction and debunk some of the most common hydration myths.

Myth #1: If You're Not Thirsty, You're Not Dehydrated

This one's a classic, and it's about as accurate as a weather forecast from a groundhog. While thirst is your body's natural signal for needing fluids, it's not always the most reliable indicator. By the time you feel thirsty, you might already be mildly dehydrated. Think of thirst as your body's "check engine" light – it's a warning sign, but it doesn't mean everything is fine until the light comes on.

To stay ahead of the dehydration curve, aim to drink water throughout the day, even if you don't feel thirsty. Remember, prevention is always better than cure.

Myth #2: All Fluids Count Towards Your Daily Water Intake

While it's true that other beverages like juice, tea, and even coffee contain water, they're not necessarily the best way to hydrate your body. Many of these drinks contain sugar, caffeine, or other diuretics that can actually dehydrate you. Think of it like trying to fill a leaky bucket – you might be putting water in, but it's also leaking out faster than you can replenish it.

Water is always the best choice for hydration because it's calorie-free, caffeine-free, and doesn't contain any diuretics. So, while it's okay to enjoy other beverages in moderation, make sure water is your primary source of hydration.

Myth #3: You Can Drink Too Much Water

This myth is a bit of a paradox. While it's technically possible to drink too much water (a condition called hyponatremia), it's incredibly rare and usually only occurs in extreme situations like endurance athletes over hydrating during long events. For the average person, it's virtually impossible to drink too much water.

Your kidneys are incredibly efficient at filtering excess water out of your system, so as long as you're not chugging gallons of water at a time, you're unlikely to overdo it. Listen to your body's thirst cues and drink when you're thirsty, and you'll be just fine.

Myth #4: Caffeinated Beverages Dehydrate You

This one's a bit of a mixed bag. While caffeine is a mild diuretic, meaning it can increase urine production, the overall effect on hydration is negligible. Studies have shown that moderate caffeine consumption (up to 400mg per day, or about 4 cups of coffee) doesn't significantly dehydrate you.

However, if you're guzzling coffee all day long or relying on energy drinks for your caffeine fix, you might want to consider adding some extra water to your routine to counteract the diuretic effect.

Myth #5: Sports Drinks Are Always Better Than Water

This myth is often perpetuated by marketing campaigns and flashy commercials. While sports drinks can be beneficial for athletes during prolonged or intense exercise, they're not always necessary for the average person.

Sports drinks contain electrolytes like sodium and potassium, which are lost through sweat. But unless you're sweating buckets or exercising for more than an hour, plain water is usually sufficient to replenish your fluids.

Myth #6: Bottled Water is Always Better Than Tap Water

This myth is often fueled by concerns about tap water quality and safety. While bottled water can be a convenient option, it's not always superior to tap water. In fact, in many areas, tap water is just as safe and clean as bottled water, and it's much more environmentally friendly.

If you're concerned about the quality of your tap water, consider using a filter or purchasing a reusable water bottle with a built-in filter. This will give you peace of mind while also reducing plastic waste.

Myth #7: You Can Survive on Metabolic Water Alone

This myth is not only false but also potentially dangerous. Metabolic water is the water produced by your body during metabolic processes, but it's not enough to sustain you. You need to drink water to replenish fluids lost through sweat, urine, and even breathing.

Attempting to survive on metabolic water alone is like trying to run a car on fumes – it's not sustainable and will eventually lead to dehydration and other health problems.

Myth #8: You Should Drink 8 Glasses of Water a Day

We've already touched on this one, but it's worth repeating: the "8x8 rule" is not a universal truth. Your individual water needs will vary depending on your activity level, climate, and overall health.

Instead of focusing on a specific number, pay attention to your body's thirst cues and drink water throughout the day. If you're feeling thirsty, that's your body's way of telling you it needs more fluids.

SIP SMARTER: CHOOSING THE BEST WATER FOR YOUR HEALTH

Alright, water warriors, prepare to become connoisseurs of hydration! We're about to embark on a taste test (well, not literally) of the different types of water available, from humble tap water to fancy bottled varieties. Get ready to discover the nuances of taste, purity, and health benefits as we explore the wide world of water options and help you choose the best one for your needs.

Tap Water: The Unsung Hero

Let's start with the most accessible and affordable option: tap water. While it might not have the marketing budget of bottled brands, tap water is a safe, convenient, and often overlooked source of hydration. In most developed countries, tap water is rigorously tested and regulated to ensure its safety and quality.

Pros of Tap Water:

- Affordable: It's practically free!
- Convenient: Available in your home, workplace, and most public places.
- Environmentally Friendly: Reduces plastic waste associated with bottled water.

Cons of Tap Water:

- Taste and Odor: Depending on your location, tap water might have a chlorine taste or odor.
- Potential Contaminants: While rare, tap water can sometimes contain trace amounts of contaminants like lead or pesticides.

Filtering Out the Doubts:

If you're concerned about the taste or quality of your tap water, consider using a water filter. There are various types of filters available, from simple pitchers to whole-house systems, that can remove impurities and improve the taste of your water.

Bottled Water: The Convenient Choice

Next up, we have bottled water, the ubiquitous beverage that's become a staple in many households and on-the-go lifestyles. While convenient, bottled water comes with its own set of pros and cons.

Pros of Bottled Water:

- Convenience: Readily available in a variety of sizes and brands.
- Taste: Often perceived as having a cleaner, crisper taste than tap water.
- Variety: You can choose from different types of bottled water, like spring water, purified water, or mineral water.

Cons of Bottled Water:

- Cost: It can get expensive over time.
- Environmental Impact: Contributes to plastic waste and pollution.
- Not Always Superior: Bottled water isn't necessarily healthier or safer than tap water.

Filtered vs. Bottled: The Showdown

So, which one is better for your health: filtered tap water or bottled water? The answer depends on your individual preferences and priorities.

If you're looking for the most affordable and environmentally friendly option, filtered tap water is the way to go. But if convenience and taste are your top priorities, bottled water might be a better choice.

The important thing is to choose a water source that you feel good about and that meets your hydration needs. And remember, no matter what type of water you choose, the most important thing is to drink enough of it!

Other Water Options: Exploring the Alternatives

While tap and bottled water are the most common choices, there are a few other options worth exploring:

- Sparkling Water: If you crave fizz, sparkling water can be a healthy alternative to sugary sodas. Just be sure to choose brands that don't contain added sugar or artificial sweeteners.
- Mineral Water: This type of water comes from natural springs and contains various minerals, including calcium, magnesium, and potassium. Some people believe mineral water has additional health benefits, but more research is needed.
- Alkaline Water: This water has a higher pH level than regular water and is often marketed as having health benefits. However, there's limited scientific evidence to support these claims.

Choosing Your Hydration Champion

Ultimately, the best water for you is the one that you enjoy drinking and that fits your lifestyle and budget. Whether you prefer tap water, bottled water, or something else entirely, the most important thing is to stay hydrated and reap the countless benefits of this amazing liquid.

So, go forth, water warriors, and choose your hydration champion!

FLAVOR FUSION: INFUSING WATER WITH FRUITS AND HERBS

Alright, water warriors, it's time to unleash your inner mixologist! While plain water is undeniably refreshing and healthy, let's face it – sometimes it can get a little boring. But fear not, hydration enthusiasts, because we're about to embark on a flavor-filled adventure, transforming your ordinary water into a tantalizing taste sensation. Get ready to discover the art of infusing water with fruits, herbs, and spices, and turn your hydration routine into a delightful daily ritual.

Why Infuse? The Flavor Factor

Let's be honest – sometimes water can feel a bit bland. And while it's always the healthiest choice, the lack of flavor can make it hard to reach for the water bottle when other, more tempting beverages are calling your name. But here's the good news: infusing your water with natural ingredients is a simple, healthy, and delicious way to up your hydration game.

Not only does infusing water add a burst of flavor, but it can also provide additional health benefits. Fruits, herbs, and spices are packed with vitamins, minerals, and antioxidants that can boost your immune system, aid digestion, and even help you glow from the inside out.

The Flavor Fusion Formula: Simple Steps for Infusing Water

Ready to create your own hydration masterpieces? Here's the basic formula for infusing water:

1. Choose Your Ingredients: The possibilities are endless! Experiment with different fruits, herbs, and spices to find your favorite flavor combinations. Some popular choices include:

- Fruits: Citrus fruits (lemons, limes, oranges), berries (strawberries, raspberries, blueberries), cucumbers, watermelon, melon
- Herbs: Mint, basil, rosemary, cilantro, lavender
- Spices: Ginger, cinnamon, cloves, cardamom

2. **Prep Your Ingredients:** Wash and chop your fruits and herbs. For spices, you can use whole pieces or ground them for a stronger flavor.
3. **Combine and Infuse:** Add your ingredients to a pitcher of water and let it infuse for at least 30 minutes, or up to several hours in the refrigerator. The longer it infuses, the stronger the flavor will be.
4. **Sip and Savor:** Pour yourself a glass of your delicious infused water and enjoy! You can refill the pitcher with water several times before the flavor starts to fade.

Flavor Inspiration: Recipes for Refreshment

Need some inspiration? Here are a few delicious infused water recipes to get you started:

- **Citrus Burst:** Combine sliced lemons, limes, and oranges for a refreshing, zesty drink.
- **Berry Bliss:** Add a handful of mixed berries to your water for a sweet and tangy treat.
- **Cucumber Cooler:** Slice up some cucumbers and add a few sprigs of mint for a spa-like experience.
- **Ginger Zing:** Grate some fresh ginger and add it to your water for a spicy kick that can also aid digestion.
- **Tropical Twist:** Combine pineapple chunks, mango slices, and a few sprigs of cilantro for a taste of the tropics.

Bonus Tip: For an extra refreshing twist, try freezing some of your infused water into ice cubes and adding them to your drinks.

Infusing Your Way to Hydration Happiness

Infusing your water is a fun and creative way to make hydration more enjoyable. It's also a great way to experiment with different flavors and find combinations that you love. So, go ahead and unleash your inner mixologist – your taste buds (and your body) will thank you!

Remember, staying hydrated is essential for your health and well-being, but it doesn't have to be boring. With a little creativity and a few simple ingredients, you can transform your water into a delicious and refreshing beverage that you'll actually look forward to drinking. So, what are you waiting for? Get infusing and start sipping your way to hydration happiness!

WATER ON THE GO: STAYING HYDRATED THROUGHOUT YOUR DAY

Water warriors, it's time to take our hydration habits on the road! Let's face it, life doesn't always happen within arm's reach of a water cooler. Whether you're commuting, running errands, traveling, or simply juggling a busy schedule, staying hydrated on the go can be a challenge. But fear not, thirst-quenchers, because we're about to equip you with the tools, tips, and tricks to keep your hydration levels high, no matter where your adventures take you.

Hydration Obstacles: The Challenges of Staying Hydrated On the Go

Before we dive into our hydration toolkit, let's acknowledge the common obstacles that can derail our best intentions:

- **The Convenience Conundrum:** Let's be honest, sometimes it's just easier to grab a sugary soda or a cup of coffee than to hunt down a water fountain or refill your reusable bottle.
- **The Forgetfulness Factor:** Life gets busy, and sometimes we simply forget to drink water until we're parched and our heads are pounding.
- **The Temptation Trap:** Vending machines, coffee shops, and convenience stores are filled with tempting beverages that can easily distract us from our hydration goals.

Hydration Heroes: Tools for On-the-Go Hydration

But fear not, water warriors, because we've got your back! Here are a few essential tools to help you stay hydrated no matter where your day takes you:

1. The Reusable Water Bottle: This is your hydration

sidekick, your trusty companion on your quest for optimal hydration. Choose a bottle that's leak-proof, easy to clean, and fits comfortably in your bag or cup holder. Bonus points if it has a built-in filter to remove impurities from tap water on the go.

2. The Hydration App: In the age of smartphones, there's an app for everything, including hydration. These handy apps can track your water intake, remind you to drink, and even gamify the process to make it more fun.

3. The Portable Water Filter: If you're worried about the quality of tap water in public places or while traveling, a portable water filter can be a lifesaver. These compact devices can remove bacteria, viruses, and other contaminants, giving you peace of mind and ensuring access to clean water wherever you are.

4. The Infused Water Bottle: If plain water isn't your jam, an infused water bottle can be a game-changer. These bottles have a built-in infuser basket where you can add your favorite fruits, herbs, or spices to create delicious and refreshing flavored water.

Hydration Hacks: Tips and Tricks for Staying Hydrated On the Go

Now that you're armed with your hydration toolkit, let's dive into some practical tips and tricks for staying hydrated throughout your day:

1. Start Your Day with Water: Kickstart your hydration by drinking a glass of water first thing in the morning. This will help replenish fluids lost overnight and set you up for a hydrated day.

2. Keep Water Within Reach: Whether you're at your desk, in your car, or running errands, always have a water bottle on hand. Make it a habit to sip on water throughout the day, even if you don't feel thirsty.

3. Set Reminders: Use your phone's alarm or a hydration app to remind you to drink water regularly. You can

even get creative with your reminders, like setting a "hydration happy hour" or a "water break dance party."

4. Pre-Hydrate Before Activities: If you know you'll be out and about, make sure to drink plenty of water beforehand. This will give your body a head start and help prevent dehydration later on.

5. Choose Water-Rich Foods: In addition to drinking water, you can also get hydration from water-rich fruits and vegetables like watermelon, cucumbers, and berries. These snacks can be a refreshing and hydrating alternative to processed foods.

6. Limit Dehydrating Beverages: While it's okay to enjoy coffee, tea, or other beverages in moderation, be mindful of their potential dehydrating effects. Try to alternate these drinks with water throughout the day.

7. Pack Your Hydration Essentials: When you're heading out, make sure to pack your water bottle, a portable water filter (if needed), and any other hydration tools you might need.

Remember, staying hydrated on the go is a marathon, not a sprint. It requires planning, preparation, and a little bit of creativity. But with the right tools and strategies, you can ensure that your body gets the hydration it needs, no matter where your adventures take you.

HYDRATION FOR ATHLETES: WATER WARRIORS, LEVEL UP!

Calling all athletes, gym rats, and weekend warriors! If you're someone who loves to push your body to its limits, this chapter is your playbook for maximizing performance and recovery through optimal hydration. Whether you're a marathon runner, a weightlifter, a yogi, or a casual exerciser, water is your secret weapon for achieving peak athletic prowess. So, grab your sweatbands (and your trusty water bottle, of course) as we dive into the world of hydration for athletes.

Why Athletes Need More H_2O: The Sweat Factor

Let's face it, athletes sweat...a lot. And with all that perspiration comes a significant loss of fluids and electrolytes. This is why staying hydrated is absolutely crucial for athletes of all levels. When you're sweating buckets, your body needs more water to replenish lost fluids, regulate temperature, and maintain optimal performance.

Think of your body like a high-performance engine. When it's running low on coolant (aka water), it starts to overheat, sputter, and eventually break down. The same goes for your body during exercise. Without enough water, your muscles fatigue faster, your heart rate increases, and your cognitive function can suffer.

Dehydration Dangers: Game Over for Athletes

For athletes, dehydration isn't just a minor inconvenience – it can be a major setback. Here are some of the ways dehydration can sabotage your athletic performance:

- Decreased Endurance: When you're dehydrated, your blood volume decreases, making it harder for your heart to pump oxygen and nutrients to your working muscles. This can lead to fatigue, weakness, and a shortened workout.

- Muscle Cramps: Dehydration can also trigger muscle cramps, those painful involuntary contractions that can stop you in your tracks.
- Heat Illness: In severe cases, dehydration can lead to heat exhaustion or heatstroke, which are serious medical conditions that require immediate attention.

Hydration Strategies for Athletic Success

So, how can you ensure you're getting enough H_2O to fuel your athletic endeavors? Here are some expert tips:

1. Pre-Game Hydration: Don't wait until you're thirsty to start hydrating. Begin drinking water several hours before your workout or competition to ensure your body is properly hydrated from the start.
2. Hydration During Exercise: Sip on water regularly throughout your workout to replace fluids lost through sweat. A good rule of thumb is to drink 7-10 ounces of water every 10-20 minutes of exercise. If you're exercising for more than an hour or in hot weather, consider a sports drink containing electrolytes to replenish lost sodium and potassium.
3. Post-Workout Recovery: Continue to hydrate after your workout to replenish fluids and aid in muscle recovery. Aim to drink 16-24 ounces of water for every pound of body weight lost during exercise.
4. Listen to Your Body: Thirst is your body's natural signal for needing fluids. Don't ignore it! If you're feeling thirsty, drink up, even if it's not during your scheduled hydration breaks.
5. Know the Signs of Dehydration: Be aware of the symptoms of dehydration, such as dry mouth, fatigue, headache, and dark urine. If you experience any of these signs, stop your activity and rehydrate immediately.

The Hydration Edge: Elevate Your Athletic Game

Staying hydrated isn't just about preventing dehydration – it's about optimizing your performance and reaching your full potential as an athlete. When you're properly hydrated, you'll have more energy, endurance, and stamina, allowing you to train harder, recover faster, and ultimately achieve your athletic goals.

So, water warriors, make hydration a priority in your athletic journey. It's the simplest, most effective way to fuel your body, protect your health, and unleash your inner champion.

THE HYDRATION HACK: MAKING WATER IRRESISTIBLE

Alright, water warriors, it's time for a hydration makeover! While we've established that water is the ultimate elixir for your health and well-being, let's face it – sometimes plain water can feel a bit... meh. If you're struggling to meet your daily water intake goals, or simply looking to add a little pizzazz to your hydration routine, this chapter is for you. We're about to unleash a torrent of tips, tricks, and hacks to make water not only essential, but downright irresistible.

The Anti-Blah Blues: Conquering the Plain Water Plateau

Let's be honest, plain water can sometimes feel about as exciting as watching paint dry. But fear not, hydration enthusiasts! There are countless ways to jazz up your H_2O and make it a beverage you actually crave. Here are a few strategies to turn your water from "blah" to "ah-mazing":

1. Infuse Your Imagination: We've already explored the wonderful world of infused water in Chapter 16, but it bears repeating. Adding fruits, herbs, or spices to your water can transform it from a boring beverage to a flavor-packed fiesta. Think of it as a spa day for your taste buds!

2. Chill Out: Sometimes, all it takes to make water more appealing is a little chill. Invest in a reusable water bottle that keeps your water icy cold, or add a few ice cubes to your glass for a refreshing kick.

3. Sip in Style: Ditch the boring plastic cup and upgrade to a fancy glass or a fun water bottle with a funky design. You'll be surprised how much more enjoyable it is to

drink water when it's served in a stylish vessel.

4. Make it a Ritual: Transform your water intake into a daily ritual. Set aside specific times to drink water, like first thing in the morning, before meals, or during breaks. You can even create a hydration mantra or affirmation to make it more fun.

5. Track Your Triumphs: There's something incredibly satisfying about checking things off a list. Use a water-tracking app or simply mark your progress on a calendar to visualize your hydration goals and celebrate your successes.

6. Join the Hydration Challenge: Enlist a friend, family member, or coworker to join you on your hydration journey. You can set goals together, share tips and recipes, and even compete to see who can drink the most water.

7. Reward Yourself: Treat yourself to a small reward each time you reach a hydration milestone. It could be anything from a new water bottle to a relaxing bath with essential oils.

8. Gamify Your Goals: Turn your hydration into a game! There are apps and online challenges that can help you track your water intake and compete with others.

9. Flavor Your Fizz: If you love bubbly drinks, try sparkling water instead of sugary sodas. You can even add a splash of juice or a few slices of fruit for extra flavor.

10. Get Creative: Don't be afraid to experiment! Try adding a pinch of salt to your water for a natural electrolyte boost, or mix in a tablespoon of apple cider vinegar for a

digestive aid.

Hydration Hacks for Every Lifestyle:

Here are a few more ideas to make water irresistible, tailored to different lifestyles:

- Busy Bees: Keep a water bottle on your desk and refill it throughout the day. Set alarms to remind you to drink.
- Fitness Fanatics: Invest in a hydration belt or backpack to carry water with you on the go. Add electrolytes to your water if you're sweating heavily.
- Travelers: Pack a reusable water bottle and refill it at water fountains or filtered water stations. Research safe drinking water options at your destination.
- Foodies: Experiment with infused water recipes using your favorite fruits, herbs, and spices. Add a splash of water to your smoothies or soups for extra hydration.

The Bottom Line:

Staying hydrated doesn't have to be a chore. With a little creativity and a willingness to experiment, you can transform water into a delicious and enjoyable beverage that you'll actually look forward to drinking. So, go forth, water warriors, and make hydration your new obsession!

WATER AND YOUR WALLET:
THE COST-EFFECTIVE
HEALTH CHOICE

Alright, water warriors, it's time to talk about something we all love: saving money! While we've been focused on the countless health benefits of water, it's important to acknowledge that it's also a budget-friendly choice. In fact, choosing water over sugary drinks and other beverages can significantly impact your wallet, leaving you with more money to spend on things that truly matter (like that new pair of running shoes you've been eyeing). So, grab your piggy bank (and your water bottle, of course) as we dive into the economics of hydration and discover how water can be your wallet's best friend.

The Costly Consequences of Sugary Drinks

Let's start by looking at the financial impact of choosing sugary drinks over water. Those tempting sodas, juices, energy drinks, and fancy coffee concoctions might seem like harmless indulgences, but they can quickly add up, both in terms of calories and cash.

Consider this: a 20-ounce bottle of soda can cost upwards of $2, and that's just for one serving! If you're indulging in sugary drinks multiple times a day, you could be spending a small fortune on empty calories that offer no nutritional value. Over time, this can lead to weight gain, health problems, and a serious dent in your wallet.

Water: The Budget-Friendly Beverage

On the other hand, water is practically free. If you're drinking tap water, you're essentially paying pennies per gallon for a beverage that's not only healthy but also refreshing and delicious (especially when infused with fruits and herbs). Even if you prefer bottled water, it's still a more affordable option than most sugary drinks.

Think of all the things you could do with the money you save by switching to water:

- **Invest in your health:** You could use that money to buy healthy groceries, sign up for a gym membership, or invest in other wellness activities.
- **Save for a rainy day:** Putting that extra cash into a savings account can provide peace of mind and financial security.
- **Treat yourself:** Why not splurge on a massage, a weekend getaway, or that new pair of running shoes you've been eyeing?

The Hidden Costs of Dehydration: More Than Just Money

While the financial impact of sugary drinks is obvious, there are also hidden costs associated with dehydration. When you're not drinking enough water, you're more likely to experience fatigue, headaches, and other health problems that can affect your productivity, energy levels, and overall quality of life.

These hidden costs can manifest in various ways:

- **Decreased Productivity:** Dehydration can lead to fatigue, difficulty concentrating, and decreased cognitive function, all of which can negatively impact your performance at work or school.
- **Increased Healthcare Costs:** Chronic dehydration can contribute to health problems like kidney stones, urinary tract infections, and constipation, which can lead to increased healthcare costs.
- **Missed Opportunities:** When you're feeling sluggish and unwell due to dehydration, you might miss out on social events, exercise opportunities, or other activities that bring you joy and fulfillment.

Hydration: A Smart Investment in Your Health and Wealth

By choosing water over sugary drinks, you're not just saving money – you're investing in your health and well-being. Water is the most natural, affordable, and effective way to stay hydrated, support your body's functions, and prevent a host of health problems.

So, the next time you're tempted to reach for a sugary drink, consider the cost – both to your wallet and your health. Choose water instead, and watch your savings (and your health) flourish!

WATER AROUND THE WORLD: CULTURAL HYDRATION PRACTICES

Water warriors, pack your virtual passports because we're embarking on a global hydration adventure! In this chapter, we're ditching the science lab and venturing into the vibrant world of different cultures to explore their unique relationships with water. Get ready to discover fascinating traditions, rituals, and beliefs surrounding hydration from every corner of the globe. Who knows, you might even find inspiration for your own water-loving rituals!

Hydration: A Universal Need, A Cultural Expression

While the need for water is universal, the way we consume and celebrate this life-giving liquid varies greatly across cultures. From ancient rituals to modern-day customs, water has played a central role in human societies for centuries, shaping our beliefs, traditions, and even our identities. Let's take a whirlwind tour of some of the most fascinating cultural hydration practices from around the world:

Japan: The Art of Tea Ceremonies

In Japan, the simple act of drinking tea is elevated to an art form. Tea ceremonies, known as "chanoyu," are elaborate rituals steeped in history and tradition. These ceremonies involve the meticulous preparation and presentation of matcha, a finely ground green tea powder, and are often accompanied by traditional sweets and Zen-like mindfulness.

While tea ceremonies might seem a world away from your morning cup of joe, they offer a beautiful example of how water can be transformed into a cultural experience that nourishes both body and soul.

India: The Sacred Ganges River

In India, the Ganges River is not just a body of water – it's a sacred entity, a goddess personified. Hindus believe that bathing in the Ganges can cleanse them of sins and purify their souls. Millions of pilgrims flock to the river each year to partake in this holy ritual, often carrying water from the Ganges back to their homes as a blessed offering.

While the scientific benefits of bathing in the Ganges might be debatable, the cultural significance of this practice is undeniable. It's a powerful reminder of how water can be a source of spiritual connection and cultural identity.

Mexico: Agua Frescas - A Refreshing Tradition

In Mexico, hot summer days are often accompanied by the refreshing taste of "agua fresca," a traditional beverage made with water, fruit, and a touch of sweetness. These thirst-quenching drinks come in a variety of flavors, from tangy tamarind to sweet watermelon, and are often enjoyed as a refreshing snack or a light dessert.

Agua fresca is more than just a tasty beverage – it's a cultural tradition that celebrates the abundance of fresh fruits and the importance of staying hydrated in hot weather. It's also a reminder that hydration can be delicious and fun!

Finland: Sauna Culture - Sweating It Out

In Finland, sauna culture is deeply ingrained in the national identity. Saunas are not just a place to get clean – they're a social gathering spot, a place for relaxation and rejuvenation, and even a sacred space for some. The Finnish sauna experience typically involves alternating between hot, dry heat and cold plunges in a lake or pool, followed by a period of rest and rehydration.

While the extreme temperatures of a Finnish sauna might not be for everyone, there's no denying the benefits of sweating it out and rehydrating afterward. It's a cultural practice that highlights the importance of water for both physical and mental well-being.

Your Hydration Passport: Exploring Global Traditions

These are just a few examples of the diverse and fascinating ways that different cultures approach hydration. From ancient rituals to modern-day customs, water plays a central role in human societies around the world. By exploring these traditions, we can gain a deeper appreciation for the cultural significance of water and find inspiration for our own hydration practices.

So, the next time you reach for your water bottle, take a moment to reflect on the rich history and diverse traditions associated with this life-giving liquid. And who knows, you might even be inspired to create your own hydration ritual, whether it's a simple morning tea ceremony or a refreshing afternoon agua fresca.

YOUR WATER'S IMPACT: THE RIPPLE EFFECT OF YOUR CHOICES

Alright, water warriors, time to put on our environmental hats and dive into a topic that's close to all our hearts (and planet!): the environmental impact of our water choices. We've talked about how water affects our bodies and minds, but now it's time to zoom out and see how our hydration habits ripple through the world around us. Get ready to discover the hidden consequences of your water choices, and learn how you can make a positive impact with every sip.

The Water Footprint: More Than Meets the Eye

Before we get into the specifics, let's talk about the concept of a "water footprint." Just like your carbon footprint measures your impact on the environment through greenhouse gas emissions, your water footprint measures the total amount of water used to produce the goods and services you consume.

This includes not just the water you drink, but also the water used to grow your food, manufacture your clothes, and power your home. It's a complex calculation, but the bottom line is that our everyday choices have a significant impact on the world's water resources.

Bottled Water Blues: The Plastic Problem

Let's start with the elephant in the room: bottled water. While convenient and often perceived as a healthier option, bottled water comes with a hefty environmental price tag.

- Plastic Pollution: The production of plastic water bottles requires vast amounts of fossil fuels and energy. And once those bottles are empty, they often end up in landfills or, worse, our oceans, where they can take centuries to decompose and harm marine life.

- Carbon Footprint: The transportation of bottled water from source to consumer also contributes to greenhouse gas emissions, further exacerbating climate change.
- Water Waste: Believe it or not, it takes more water to produce a bottle of water than it does to fill it! The bottled water industry uses an estimated 17 million barrels of oil each year to produce plastic bottles, enough to fuel 1.3 million cars for a year.

Tap Water Triumphs: A Sustainable Solution

So, what's the alternative? Tap water, of course! In most developed countries, tap water is a safe, affordable, and environmentally friendly option. By choosing tap water over bottled water, you can significantly reduce your water footprint and help protect our planet.

Filtered Water: The Best of Both Worlds

If you're concerned about the taste or quality of your tap water, consider using a filter. This will not only improve the taste and remove impurities, but it will also reduce your environmental impact by eliminating the need for plastic bottles.

Beyond the Bottle: Other Ways to Reduce Your Water Footprint

But reducing your water footprint goes beyond just choosing tap over bottled water. Here are a few other ways you can make a difference:

- Reduce Water Waste: Be mindful of your water usage at home and work. Fix leaky faucets, take shorter showers, and only run the dishwasher and washing machine with full loads.
- Eat Less Meat: The production of meat requires a significant amount of water. By reducing your meat consumption, you can lower your water footprint and contribute to a more

sustainable food system.

- Choose Sustainable Products: Support companies that prioritize water conservation and sustainable practices. Look for products with eco-friendly certifications or those made with recycled materials.
- Get Involved: Support organizations that are working to protect our water resources and advocate for policies that promote water conservation.

The Ripple Effect: Your Choices Matter

Remember, every drop counts! Your individual choices might seem small, but collectively they can have a huge impact on our planet's water resources. By making conscious choices about your water consumption, you can reduce your water footprint, conserve this precious resource, and contribute to a healthier planet for future generations.

So, let's raise a glass (of tap water, of course!) to a more sustainable future. Cheers to making a difference, one sip at a time!

BEYOND THE BOTTLE: WATER CONSERVATION TIPS FOR A THIRSTY PLANET

Alright, water warriors, time to channel your inner eco-warrior and explore the world of water conservation! We've talked about the importance of hydration for our bodies and the environmental impact of our water choices, but now it's time to take action. Get ready to discover practical tips and tricks for conserving water at home, work, and play, because every drop counts when it comes to protecting this precious resource.

Water Woes: The Global Water Crisis

Before we dive into our water-saving strategies, let's take a moment to acknowledge the global water crisis. While water covers about 71% of our planet's surface, only a tiny fraction of that is freshwater that we can use for drinking, sanitation, and agriculture. And with a growing population and increasing demand for water, this precious resource is becoming scarcer by the day.

The consequences of water scarcity are far-reaching, affecting everything from food production to public health to economic stability. Droughts, water pollution, and inadequate sanitation are just a few of the challenges facing communities around the world. But the good news is that we can all make a difference by taking simple steps to conserve water in our daily lives.

Water-Saving Superheroes: Everyday Actions, Extraordinary Impact

Think of yourself as a water-saving superhero, armed with the power to make a difference with every flush, shower, and laundry load. Here are some simple yet effective tips for conserving water at home:

1. Fix those leaks: A leaky faucet might seem like a minor annoyance, but it can waste a surprising amount of water over time. Get those leaks fixed ASAP to save water (and money on your water bill!).
2. Upgrade your appliances: Older toilets, showerheads, and washing machines can be water guzzlers. Consider upgrading to high-efficiency models that use less water without sacrificing performance. It's an investment that will pay off in the long run, both for your wallet and the planet.
3. Mindful showers: Long, luxurious showers might feel amazing, but they're not so great for the environment. Challenge yourself to shorten your showers by a few minutes, or try taking a "navy shower," where you turn off the water while lathering up.
4. Full loads only: When it comes to washing machines and dishwashers, only run them when they're full. This will save both water and energy.
5. Don't let it run: Turn off the faucet while brushing your teeth, washing your hands, or shaving. It might seem like a small thing, but those minutes add up over time.
6. Water-wise landscaping: Choose drought-tolerant plants for your garden, water your lawn early in the morning or late in the evening to minimize evaporation, and consider using a rain barrel to collect rainwater for irrigation.
7. Think before you flush: Don't use your toilet as a trash can. Only flush when necessary, and consider installing a low-flow toilet to reduce water usage.

Water Warriors at Work: Conservation in the Workplace

But water conservation doesn't stop at home. You can also make a difference at work by:

- Reporting leaks and malfunctions: If you see a leaky faucet or toilet at work, don't hesitate to report it to maintenance.

- Encouraging water-wise practices: Talk to your coworkers and employer about ways to conserve water in the workplace.
- Choosing sustainable options: If your workplace provides bottled water, advocate for switching to filtered tap water or installing water fountains.

Water Conservation: A Global Responsibility

Remember, water conservation is not just a personal responsibility, it's a global one. By making small changes in our daily lives, we can collectively make a big impact on our planet's water resources. So, let's all do our part to protect this precious resource and ensure a sustainable future for generations to come.

As the saying goes, "Every drop counts." So, water warriors, let's make every drop count towards a healthier planet!

THE 21-DAY WATER CHALLENGE: A SPLASH OF FUN ON YOUR HYDRATION JOURNEY

Water warriors, it's time to put all that water wisdom into action! We've explored the science, the benefits, and the hacks, but now it's time to challenge ourselves and transform our hydration habits for good. Get ready to embark on a 21-day water adventure that will leave you feeling refreshed, revitalized, and ready to conquer the world (or at least your thirst).

Why 21 Days? The Habit-Forming Magic

You might be wondering, why 21 days? Well, research suggests that it takes about 21 days to form a new habit. By committing to a 21-day water challenge, you're not just drinking more water for a short period – you're creating a sustainable change that will benefit you for years to come.

Think of it like training for a marathon. You don't just wake up one day and run 26.2 miles. You start with shorter distances, gradually increasing your mileage over time until you're ready for the big race. The same goes for hydration. This 21-day challenge is your training ground for developing a lifelong habit of drinking plenty of water.

The Challenge: Simple Yet Powerful

The rules of the challenge are simple:

1. Drink at least eight 8-ounce glasses of water per day. This is a good starting point for most people, but you can adjust the amount based on your individual needs and the factors we discussed in Chapter 13.
2. Track your progress. Use a water-tracking app, a journal, or simply mark your progress on a calendar. Seeing your

daily achievements can be incredibly motivating!

3. Get creative! Don't be afraid to experiment with infused water, try different types of water, or set fun hydration goals for yourself. The key is to make it enjoyable and sustainable.

4. Don't give up! There might be days when you fall short of your goal, but don't beat yourself up about it. Just get back on track the next day and keep going. Remember, it's a journey, not a race.

Beyond the Basics: Extra Challenges for the Overachievers

If you're feeling ambitious, here are a few additional challenges to spice things up:

- The Flavor Challenge: Try a new infused water recipe every day for 21 days.
- The Temperature Challenge: Experiment with different water temperatures – hot, cold, or room temperature – and see how they affect your body and taste preferences.
- The Activity Challenge: Pair your hydration with different activities each day. For example, drink water while walking, reading, or working on a creative project.

The Rewards: More Than Just Quenching Your Thirst

So, what's in it for you? Completing this 21-day water challenge can bring about a cascade of positive changes:

- Increased energy and mental clarity: You'll likely notice a significant boost in your energy levels and mental focus as your body and brain become properly hydrated.
- Improved skin health: Your skin will thank you for the extra hydration, with a noticeable improvement in its texture, tone, and overall appearance.
- Weight loss support: If you're trying to lose weight, drinking more water can help suppress your appetite, boost your metabolism, and make it easier to stick to your healthy eating plan.

- Better digestion and gut health: Water is essential for optimal digestion and a healthy gut microbiome. Say goodbye to constipation and hello to a happy tummy!
- Stronger immune system: Staying hydrated can help your body fight off infections and illnesses, keeping you feeling your best.

Remember, this challenge is not just about drinking more water; it's about creating a sustainable habit that will benefit your health and well-being for years to come.

So, are you ready to take the plunge and embark on this 21-day hydration adventure? Your body will thank you!

YOUR HYDRATION JOURNEY: A LIFELONG COMMITMENT TO WELLNESS

Water warriors, congratulations on reaching the final chapter of our hydration odyssey! We've delved into the science, the benefits, the hacks, and even the cultural quirks of water consumption. Now, it's time to reflect on everything we've learned and embark on a lifelong journey of hydration and wellness. So, grab your trusty water bottle (it's probably your most prized possession by now) and let's celebrate your commitment to a healthier, happier you.

Hydration: More Than Just a Trend

Remember those fleeting health fads that come and go faster than a summer thunderstorm? Kale smoothies, detox teas, and whatever the latest Instagram influencer is promoting – they all have their moment in the sun, but they rarely stick around for the long haul.

But water, dear friends, is not a trend. It's a timeless, essential element of life that will never go out of style. It's the original superfood, the elixir of life, the fountain of youth – you name it, water probably has something to do with it.

Your Hydration Journey: A Personal Odyssey

Your relationship with water is unique, just like you. Maybe you're a seasoned hydration pro, guzzling down your daily quota with ease. Or perhaps you're a newbie, still struggling to remember to refill your water bottle. Wherever you are on your hydration journey, remember that it's a personal odyssey, not a race.

There will be days when you're chugging water like a fish, and there will be days when you're barely squeezing out a few sips.

That's okay! The important thing is to keep showing up, keep trying, and keep prioritizing your hydration.

The Power of Habit: Making Hydration Second Nature

The key to long-term success is to make hydration a habit, something so ingrained in your routine that you don't even have to think about it. Start by setting small, achievable goals, like drinking a glass of water first thing in the morning or carrying a water bottle with you wherever you go.

Once you've mastered the basics, you can start experimenting with different hydration hacks, like infusing your water with fruits and herbs, setting reminders on your phone, or even joining a water challenge with friends. The possibilities are endless!

Hydration: A Gift That Keeps on Giving

The benefits of staying hydrated extend far beyond just quenching your thirst. Water is a gift that keeps on giving, nourishing your body, mind, and spirit in countless ways.

By prioritizing hydration, you're not just investing in your health today – you're setting yourself up for a lifetime of vitality, energy, and well-being. So, raise a glass (of water, of course!) to your health, your happiness, and your commitment to a hydrated life.

Cheers to you, water warriors! You've made it to the end of this journey, and you're now equipped with the knowledge, tools, and inspiration to make hydration a lifelong priority. Keep sipping, keep exploring, and keep thriving!

P.S. Don't forget to share your hydration journey with friends and family. Encourage them to join the water warrior movement and spread the message of hydration for a healthier, happier world. After all, sharing is caring (and in this case, sharing water might just save the planet!).

www.ingramcontent.com/pod-product-compliance
Lightning Source LLC
Chambersburg PA
CBHW051650250726
48653CB00007B/2578